Beer Singh
Niharika Sharma
Falaknaz Khan

Analgesics, Anti-Inflammatory & Muscle Relaxants in Dentistry

Beer Singh
Niharika Sharma
Falaknaz Khan

Analgesics, Anti-Inflammatory & Muscle Relaxants in Dentistry

Pain management

LAP LAMBERT Academic Publishing

Imprint

Cover image: www.ingimage.com

Publisher:
LAP LAMBERT Academic Publishing
is a trademark of
Dodo Books Indian Ocean Ltd. and OmniScriptum S.R.L publishing group

120 High Road, East Finchley, London, N2 9ED, United Kingdom
Str. Armeneasca 28/1, office 1, Chisinau MD-2012, Republic of Moldova, Europe
Managing Directors: Ieva Konstantinova, Victoria Ursu
info@omniscriptum.com

Printed at: see last page
ISBN: 978-620-8-43500-4

Introduction

Analgesics are medications that treat your pain by reducing inflammation or changing the way your brain understands pain. Many types of analgesics are available, and they range from pills and liquids, to gels and patches you apply to your body. Some are available over the counter, and some require a prescription from your healthcare provider. Your provider can help you figure out the type of medication that's most effective for your type of pain.

The word "Drug" is derived from French word Drogue, a dry herb. According to WHO (1966), Drug is any substance or product that is used or intended to be used to modify or explore physiological systems or pathological systems for the benefit of the recipient. The subject of drug is as old as disease. Illness has been man's heritage from the beginning of his existence and the search for remedies to combat it is perhaps equally old.

Analgesics, also called painkillers, are medications that relieve different types of pain — from headaches to injuries to arthritis. Anti-inflammatory analgesics reduce inflammation, and opioid analgesics change the way the brain perceives pain. Some analgesics can be bought over the counter, others require a prescription.

Depending on the diagnosis treatment may consist of reassurance, surgery, or other interventions. Drugs are very often either the primary therapy or an adjunct to another modality (e.g. the use of unaesthetic s in patients undergoing surgery). Sometimes contact with doctor is initiated because of a public health measure (e.g. through a screening programme). Again, drug treatment is sometimes needed. Consequently, the doctors of nearly all specialties use drugs extensively, and need to understand the scientific basis on which therapeutic use is founded. A century ago, physicians had only a handful of effective drugs (e.g. morphia, quinine, ether, aspirin, and digitalis leaf) at their disposal. Thousands of potent drugs have since been introduced, and pharmaceutical chemists continue to discover new and better drugs. With advances in genetics, cellular and molecular science, it is likely that progress will accelerate a huge change in therapeutics are inevitable. Medical students and doctors in training therefore need to learn something of the principles of therapeutics, in order to prepare themselves to adapt to such change.

Nonsteroidal Anti-Inflammatory Drugs

Introduction

Salicylates and other similar agents used to treat rheumatic disease share the capacity to suppress the signs and symptoms of inflammation. These drugs also exert antipyretic and analgesic effects, but it is their anti-inflammatory properties that make them most useful in the management of disorders in which pain is related to the intensity of the inflammatory process. Since aspirin, the original NSAID, has a number of adverse effects, many other NSAIDS have been developed in attempts to improve upon aspirin`s efficacy and decrease its toxicity. Salicylates include Aspirin, Salicylamide, and Sodium Salicylate.

NSAIDS ARE GENERALLY USED IN THE FOLLOWING CONDITIONS

- Rheumatic Diseases, most are probably effective in rheumatoid arthritis,
- Seronegative Spondyloarthropathies (e.g., psoriatic arthritis and arthritis associated with inflammatory bowel disease), Osteoarthritis,

- Localized musculoskeletal syndromes (e.g., sprains and strains, low back pain), and. Gout (except tolmetin, which appears to be ineffective in gout).

Adverse effects are generally quite similar for all of the NSAIDS-

1. Central Nervous System – Headaches, tinnitus, and dizziness.
2. Cardiovascular –Fluid retention hypertension, edema, and rarely, congestive heart failure.
3. Gastrointestinal- Abdominal pain, dysplasia, nausea, vomiting, and rarely, ulcers or bleeding.
4. Hematologic- Rare thrombocytopenia, neutropenia, or even aplastic anemia.
5. Hepatic – Abnormal liver function tests and rare liver failure.
6. Pulmonary – Asthma.
7. Rashes- All types, pruritus.
8. Renal- Renal insufficiency, renal failure, hyperkalemia, and proteinuria.

Aspirin

- Aspirin`s long use and availability without prescription diminishes its glamour compared with that of the newer NSAIDS.
- Aspirin is now rarely used as an anti- inflammatory medication and will be reviewed only in terms of its antiplatelet effects (i.e., doses of 81- 325 mg once daily)
- Exerts analgesic, anti-pyretic and anti-inflammatory activity

Pharmacokinetics

- **Salicylic acid** is a simple organic acid with a pKa of 3.0.
- **Aspirin** (acetylsalicylic acid, ASA) has a pKa of 3.5.
- The salicylates are rapidly absorbed from the stomach and upper small intestine yielding a peak plasma salicylate level within 1-2 hrs.
- Aspirin is absorbed as such and is rapidly hydrolyzed (serum half-life 15 mins.) to acetic acid and salicylate by esterases in tissue and blood.
- Salicylate is nonlinearly bound to albumin.
- Alkalinization of the urine increases the rate of excretion of free salicylate and its water-soluble conjugates.

Mechanism of action

- Aspirin irreversibly inhibits platelet COX so that aspirins antiplatelet effect lasts 8-10 days.
- In other tissues, synthesis of new COX replaces the inactivated enzyme so that ordinary doses have duration of action of 6-12 hrs.

Clinical uses

- Aspirin decreases the incidence of transient ischemic attacks.
- Unstable angina
- Coronary artery thrombosis with myocardial infarction
- And thrombosis after coronary artery by - pass grafting.
- Epidemiological studies suggest that long term use of aspirin at low dosage is associated with a lower incidence of colon cancer, possibly related to its COX inhibiting effects.

Adverse effects

- In addition to the common side effects listed above, aspirins main adverse effect at anti thrombotic doses are gastric upset (intolerance) and gastric and duodenal ulcers.

- Hepatotoxicity, asthma, rashes, gastrointestinal bleeding, and renal toxicity rarely if ever occur at anti thrombotic doses.
- The antiplatelet action of aspirin contraindicates its use by patients with hemophilia.
- Although previously not recommended during pregnancy, aspirin may be valuable in treating pre-eclampsia – eclampsia.

Nonacetylated salicylates

- These drugs include magnesium choline salicylate, sodium salicylate, and salicyl salicylate.
- All nonacetylated salicylates are effective anti-inflammatory drugs although they may be fewer effective analgesics than aspirin.
- Because they are much less effective than aspirin as COX inhibitors and they do not inhibit platelet aggregation, they may be preferable when COX inhibition is undesirable such as in patients with asthma, those with bleeding tendencies, and even (under close supervision) those with renal dysfunction.
- The nonacetylated salicylates are administered in doses upto 3-4 g of salicylate a day and can be monitored using serum salicylate measurements.

COX-2 Selective Inhibitors

- COX-2 selective inhibitors, or coxibs, were developed in an attempt to inhibit prostaglandins synthesis by the COX-2 isozyme induced at sites of inflammation without affecting the action of the constitutively active 'housekeeping' COX -1 isozyme found in the gastrointestinal tract, kidneys, and platelets.
- Coxibs selectively bind to and block the active site of the COX-2 enzyme much more effectively than that of COX-1.
- COX-2 inhibitors have analgesic, antipyretic, and anti-inflammatory effects similar to those of nonselective NSAIDS but with an approximate halving of gastrointestinal adverse effects.
- Likewise, COX-2 inhibitors at usual doses have been shown to have no impact on platelet aggregation, which is mediated by thromboxane produced by the COX-1 isozyme.
- In contrast, they do inhibit COX-2 mediated prostacyclin synthesis in the vascular endothelium.
- As a result, COX-2 inhibitors do not offer the cardioprotective effects of traditional nonselective NSAIDS, which has resulted in some patients taking low dose aspirin in addition to a coxib regimen to maintain this effect.

- Unfortunately, because COX-2 is constitutively active within the kidney, recommended doses of COX-2 inhibitors cause renal toxicities similar to those associated with traditional NSAIDs.
- Clinical data have suggested a higher incidence of cardiovascular thrombotic events associated with COX-2 inhibitors such as rofecoxib and valdecoxib, resulting in their withdrawal from the market.

Celecoxib

- Celecoxib is a selective COX-2 inhibitor – about 10-20 times more selective for COX-2 than for COX-1.
- Celecoxib is associated with fewer endoscopic ulcers than most other NSAIDS.
- Probably because it is a sulfonamide, celecoxib may cause rashes.
- It does not affect platelet aggregation at usual doses.
- It interacts occasionally with warfarin as would be expected of a drug metabolized via CYP2C9.
- Adverse effects are the common toxicities listed above.

Meloxicam

- Meloxicam is an enolcarboxamide related to piroxicam that preferentially inhibits COX-2 over COX-1, particularly at its lowest therapeutic dose of 7.5 mg/d
- It is not as selective as celecoxib and may be considered "preferentially" selective rather than "highly" selective.
- It is associated with fewer clival gastrointestinal symptoms and complications than piroxicam, diclofenac, and naproxen.
- Similarly, while meloxicam is known to inhibit synthesis of thromboxane A2, even at supra therapeutic doses its blockade of thromboxane A2 does not reach levels that result in decreased in vivo platelet function.

Nonselective Cox Inhibitors

Diclofenac

- Diclofenac is a phenylacetic acid derivative that is relatively nonselective as a COX inhibitor.
- Gastrointestinal ulceration may occur less frequently than with some other NSAIDS.

- A preparation combining diclofenac and misoprostol decreases upper gastrointestinal ulceration but may result in diarrhea.
- Another combination of diclofenac and omeprazole was also effective with respect to the prevention of recurrent bleeding. But renal adverse effects were common in high-risk patients.
- Diclofenac 150 mg /d appears to impair renal blood flow and glomerular filtration rate.
- Elevation of serum aminotransferases occur more commonly with this drug than with other NSAIDs.
- A 0.1% ophthalmic preparation is recommended for prevention of post operative ophthalmic inflammation and can be used after intraocular lens implantation and strabismus surgery.
- A topical gel containing 3% diclofenac is effective for solar keratitis.
- Diclofenac in renal suppository form can be considered for preemptive analgesia and post operative nausea.

Flurbiprofen

- Flurbiprofen is a propionic acid derivative with a possibly more complex mechanism of action than other NSAIDs.

- Its (S) (-) enantiomer inhibits COX no selectively, but it has been shown in rat tissue to also affect tumor necrosis factor (TNF-) and nitric oxide synthesis.
- Hepatic metabolism is extensive, it's (R) (+) and (S) (-) enantiomers are metabolized differently, and it does not undergo chiral conversion.
- It does demonstrate enterohepatic circulation.
- Flurbiprofen is also available in a topical ophthalmic formulation for inhibition of intraoperative miosis.
- Flurbiprofen intravenously is effective for perioperative analgesia in minor ear, neck, and nose surgery and in lozenge form for sore throat.
- Although its adverse effect profile is similar to that of other NSAIDS in, most ways, flurbiprofen is also associated rarely with cogwheel rigidity, ataxia, tremor, and myoclonus.

Ibuprofen

- Ibuprofen is a simple derivative of phenyl propionic.
- In doses of about 2400 mg daily, ibuprofen is equivalent to 4 g of aspirin in anti-inflammatory effect.

- Oral ibuprofen is often prescribed in lower doses (2400 mg/d, at which it has analgesic but not anti-inflammatory efficacy.
- It is available over the counter in low- dose forms under several trade names.
- Ibuprofen is effective in closing patent Ductus arteriosus in preterm infants, with much the same efficacy and safety as indomethacin.
- The oral and intravenous are equally effective for this indication.
- A topical cream preparation appears to be absorbed into fascia and muscle, an (s) (-) formulations have been tested.
- Ibuprofen cream was more effective than placebo cream in the treatment of primary knee osteoarthritis.
- A liquid gel preparation of ibuprofen, 400mg, provides prompt relief and good overall efficacy in postsurgical dental pain.
- In comparison with indomethacin, ibuprofen decreases urine output less and also causes less fluid retention.
- The drug is relatively contraindicated in individuals with nasal polyps, angioedema, and bronchospastic reactivity to aspirin.
- Aseptic meningitis (particularly in patients with systemic lupus erythematosus), and fluid retention have been reported.
- Interaction with anticoagulants is uncommon.

- The concomitant administration ibuprofen and aspirin antagonizes the irreversible platelet inhibition induced by aspirin.
- Thus, treatment with ibuprofen in patients with increased cardiovascular risk may limit the cardioprotective effect of aspirin.
- Furthermore, the use of ibuprofen concomitantly with aspirin may decrease the total anti –inflammatory effect.
- Rare hematologic effects include agranulocytosis and aplastic anemia.

Indomethacin

- Indomethacin, introduced in 1963, is an indole derivative.
- It is a potent nonselective COX inhibitor and may also inhibit phospholipase A and C reduce neutrophil migration, and decrease T-cell and B-cell proliferation.
- It differs somewhat from other NSAIDs in its indications and toxicities.
- Indomethacin was particularly popular for gout and ankylosing spondylitis
- In addition, it has been used to accelerate closure of patent ductus arteriosus.

- Indomethacin has been tried in numerous **small or uncontrolled** trials for many other conditions, including Sweet's Syndrome, juvenile rheumatoid arthritis, pleurisy, nephritic syndrome, diabetes insipidus, urticarial vasculitis, post episiotomy pain and prophylaxis of heterotrophic ossification in arthroplasty.
- Gingival inflammation is reduced after administration of indomethacin oral rinse
- Epidural injections produce a degree of pain relief similar to that achieved with methylprednisolone in post laminectomy syndrome.
- The gastrointestinal effects may include pancreatitis.
- Headache is experienced by 15-25 % of patients and may be associated with dizziness, confusion, and depression.
- Rarely, psychosis with hallucinations has been reported.
- Seriously hematologic reactions have been noted, including thrombocytopenia and aplastic anemia.
- Renal papillary necrosis has also been observed.
- Probenecid prolongs indomethacin's half-life by inhibiting both renal and biliary clearance.

Ketorolac

- Ketorolac is an NSAID promoted for systemic use mainly as analgesic not as an anti-inflammatory drug. Although it has typical NSAID properties).
- The drug is an effective analgesic and has been successfully to replace morphine in some situations involving mild to moderate postsurgical pain.
- It is most often given intramuscularly or intravenously, but an oral dose formulation is available.
- When used with an opioid, it may decrease the opioid requirement by 25-50%.
- Toxicities are similar to those of other NSAIDs, although renal toxicity may be more common with chronic use.

Piroxicam

- Piroxicam, an oxicam, is a nonselective COX inhibitor that at high concentrations also inhibits polymorphonuclear leukocyte migration, decreases oxygen radical production, and inhibits lymphocyte function.
- Its long half-life permits once –daily dosing.

- Piroxicam is used in dosages higher than 20 mg/d, an increased incidence of peptic ulcer and bleeding is encountered.
- Epidemiologic studies suggest that this risk is as much as 9.5 times higher with piroxicam than with other NSAIDs.

Other analgesics

Acetaminophen is one of the most important drugs used in the treatment of mild to moderate pain when an anti-inflammatory effect is not necessary. Phenacetin, a prodrug that is metabolized to acetaminophen, is more toxic than its active metabolite and has no rational indications.

Acetaminophen

- Acetaminophen is the active metabolite of phenacetin and is responsible for its analgesic effect.
- It is a weak COX-1 and COX-2 inhibitor in peripheral tissues and possesses no significant anti-inflammatory effects.

Pharmacokinetics

- Acetaminophen is administered orally.
- Absorption is related to the rate of emptying, and peak blood concentrations are usually reached in 30-60 minutes.

- Acetaminophen is slightly bound to plasma proteins and is partially metabolized by hepatic microsomal enzymes and converted to acetaminophen sulfate and glucuronide, which are pharmacologically inactive.
- Less than 5% is excreted unchanged.
- A minor but highly active metabolite (N-acetyl-p-benzoquinone) is important in large doses because it is toxic to both liver and kidney.
- The half- life of acetaminophen is 2-3 hours and is relatively unaffected by renal function. With toxic doses of liver disease, the half –life may be increased twofold or more.

Indications

- Although said to be equivalent to aspirin as an analgesic and antipyretic agent, acetaminophen differs in that it lacks anti-inflammatory properties.
- It does not affect uric acid levels and lacks platelets –inhibiting properties.
- The drug is useful in mild to moderate pain such as headache, myalgia, postpartum pain, and other circumstances in which aspirin is an effective analgesic.

- Acetaminophen alone is inadequate therapy for inflammatory conditions such as rheumatoid arthritis, although it may be used as an analgesic adjunct to anti-inflammatory therapy.
- For mild analgesia, acetaminophen is the preferred drug in patients allergic to aspirin or when salicylates are poorly tolerated.
- It is preferable to aspirin in patients with hemophilia or a history of peptic ulcer and in those in whom bronchospasm is precipitated by aspirin.
- Unlike aspirin, acetaminophen does not antagonize the effects of uricosuric agents; it may be used concomitantly with probenecid in the treatment of gout.
- It is preferred to aspirin in children with viral infections.

Adverse effects

- In therapeutic doses, a mild increase in hepatic enzymes may occasionally occur in the absence of jaundice, this is reversible when the drug is withdrawn.
- With larger doses, dizziness, excitement, and disorientation can be seen.

- Ingestion of 15 g of acetaminophen may be fatal, death being caused by severe hepatotoxicity with centriolar necrosis, sometimes associated with acute renal tubular necrosis.
- Doses greater than 4-6g/d are not recommended and a history of alcoholism contraindicates even this dose.
- Early symptom of hepatic damage includes nausea, vomiting, diarrhea, and abdominal pain.
- Cases of renal damage without hepatic damage have occurred, even after usual doses of acetaminophen
- Therapy is much less satisfactory than for aspirin overdose.
- In addition to supportive therapy, the measures that have proved most useful are the provision of sulfhydryl groups in the form of acetylcysteine to neutralize the toxic metabolites.
- Hematolytic anemia and methemoglobinemia are very rare adverse events.
- Interstitial nephritis and papillary necrosis – serious complications of phenacetin- have not occurred nor has gastrointestinal bleeding.
- Caution is necessary in patients with any type of liver disease.

Dosage

Acute pain and fever may be effectively treated with 325 -500mg four times daily and proportionately less for children.

Preparations available

Nonsteroidal Anti- Inflammatory Drugs

Aspirin, acetylsalicylic acid (generic, aspirin, others)

Oral (regular, enteric coated, buffered), 81, 165, 325, 500, 650, 800 mg tablets, 81, 650, 800mg timed –or extended-release tablets

Rectal – 120, 200, 300, 600mg suppositories.

Bromfenac (Xibrom)

Ophthalmic -0.09% solution

Celecoxib (celebrix)

Oral- 50, 100, 200, 400mg capsules

Choline salicylate (Varius)

Oral- 870 mg / 5ml. liquid

Diclofenac (generic, cataflam, voltaren)

Oral- 50 mg tablets, 25, 50, 75 mg delayed –release tablet, 100mg extended –release tablets

Ophthalmic- 0.1% solution

Diflunisal (generic, dolobid)

Oral – 500 mg tablets

Etodolac (generic, iodine)

Oral- 200, 300mg capsules, 400, 500 mg tablets, 400, 500, 600 mg tablets extended-release tablets

Fenoprofen (generic, Nalfon)

Oral- 200, 300 mg capsules, 600 mg tablets.

Flurbiprofen- (Generic, Ansaid)

Oral-50, 100 mg tablets

Ophthalmic (generic, ocufen), 0.03 % solution

Ibuprofen- (generic, Motrin, Rufen, Advil, (otc), Nuprin (otc), others)

Oral- 100, 200, 400, 600, 800mg tablets, 50, 100mg chewable tablets, 200 mg capsules, 100mg/ 2.5 ml suspension, 100mg/ 5ml suspension, 40mg /ml drops

Indomethacin- (generic, indocin)

Oral- 25, 50, mg capsules, 75mg sustained –release capsules, 25mg/ 5ml suspension.

Rectal – 50 mg suppositories.

Ketoprofen – (generic, orudis)

Oral-12.5 mg tablets, 25, 50, 75 mg capsules, 100, 150, 200; mg extended-release capsules.

Ketorolac Tromethamine- (generic, Toradol)

Oral- 10mg tablets,

Parenteral 15, 30 mg /ml for IM injection

Ophthalmic- 0.4, 0.5 % solution

Magnesium salicylate (Doan's pills, Magan, Mobidin)

Oral- 545, 600 mg tablets, 467, 500, 580 mg capsules.

Meclofenamate sodium (generic)

Oral- 50, 100 mg capsules.

Mefenamic acid ;(Postal)

Oral 250 mg capsules

Meloxicam (Mobic)

Oral- 7.5, 15 mg tablets, 7.5 mg /5ml suspension

Nabumetone (generic)

Oral- 500, 750 mg tablets.

Naproxen (generic, Naprosyn, Anaprox, Aleve (otc)

oral -200, 220, 250, 375, 500 mg tablets, 375, 550 mg controlled released tablets, 375, 500mg delayed release tablets, 125mg / 5ml suspension.

Oxaprozin- (generic, Daypro)

Oral- 600mg tablets, capsules.

Piroxicam (generic, Feldene)

Oral- 10, 20 mg capsules.

Salsalate, salicylsalicylic acid (generic, Disalcid)

Oral- 500, 750 mg tablets, 500mg capsules.

Sodium salicylate (generic)

Oral- 325, 650 mg enteric –coated tablets

Sodium thiosalicylate (generic, Rexolate)

Parenteral – 50 mg/ ml for IM injection.

Sulindac (generic, Clinoril)

Oral- 150, 200mg tablets

Suprofen (profenal)

Topical – 1% ophthalmic solution

Tolmetin (generic, Tolectin)

Oral- 200, 600 mg tablets, 400 mg capsules.

Caution- one of the most important complications arising out of conventional anti-inflammatory –analgesic treatment given during dental pain, including those complicating NSAID therapy is benign peptic ulcers.

A new class of drugs (ulcer healing, G-I sedative and spasmodic) are included routinely in the general dental prescriptions containing NSAID's like the PPI (proton pump inhibitors) this includes omeprazole, lansoprazole, pantoprazole, esomeprazole, and rabeprazole. These drugs are indicated in Zollinger Ellison syndrome &erosive reflux esophagitis. These agents inhibit gastric acid secretion by blocking the hydrogen – potassium adenosine triphosphate enzyme system (the proton pump) in gastric parietal cells.

The enzyme inhibited is thought to be the terminal step in gastric acid production so both basal as well as the stimulated acid secretions are reduced. Healing rates and relief from symptoms are better than with H2 (Ranitidine, Cimetidine, Famotidine) antagonists, moreover healing occurs in patients previously shown to be unresponsive to these agents.

Opioid Analgesics

Introduction

- Morphine, the prototypical opioid agonist, has long been known to relieve severe pain with remarkable efficacy. The opium poppy is the source of crude opium from which serturner in 1803 isolated morphine, the pure alkaloid, naming it after Morpheus, the Greek god of dreams.
- It remains the standard against which all drugs that have strong analgesic action are compared. These drugs are collectively known as opioid analgesics and include not only the natural and semisynthetic alkaloid derivatives from opium but also synthetic surrogates, other opioid like drugs whose action are blockage by the non-selective antagonist naloxone, plus several endogenous peptides that interact with the different subtypes of opioid receptors.

Basic Pharmacology of the Opioid Analgesics

Source

- Opium, the source of morphine, is obtained from the poppy, Papaver somniferum and p album.

- After incision the, the poppy seed pod exudes the white substance that turns into a brown gum that is crude opium
- Opium contains many alkaloids, the principal being finer, which is present in a constriction of about 10% codeine, is synthesized commercially from morphine.

CLASSIFICATION AND CHEMISTRY

- Opioid drugs include full agonist, partial agonists, and antagonists.
- Morphine is a full agonist at the (mu) - opioid receptor, the major analgesics opioid receptor.
- In contrast, codeine function as a partial, (or "Weak") – receptor agonist
- Other opioid receptor subtypes include, (delta) and (Kappa) receptors. Simple substitution of an allyl group on the nitrogen of the full agonist morphine plus addition of single hydroxyl group result in naloxone, a strong receptor antagonist.
- Some opioids, e.g., nalbuhpine, are capable of producing an agonist (or partial agonist) effect at one opioid receptor sub type and an antagonist effect at another.

- Chemically, the opioid derived from opium are phenanthrene derivatives and include four or more fused rings, while most of the synthetic opioid are simpler molecules.

Mechanism of action of opioid analgesics

- Opioid agonists produce analgesia by binding to specific G protein-coupled receptors that are located in brain and spinal cord regions involved in the transmission and modulation of pain). Some effects may be mediated by opioid receptors on peripheral sensory nerve endings.
- At the molecular level, opioid receptors form a family of proteins that physically couple to G proteins and through this interaction affect ion channel gating, modulate intracellular Ca+ 2 disposition, and alter protein phosphorylation.
- The opioids have two well –established direct G protein – coupled actions on neurons.
- They close voltage –gated Ca+2 channels on presynaptic nerve terminals and thereby reduce transmitter release, and
- They hyperpolarize and thus inhibit postsynaptic neurons by opening K+ channels.

- The presynaptic action –depressed transmitter release – has been demonstrated for release – has been demonstrated for release of a large number of neurotransmitters including glutamate, the principle excitatory amino acid released from nociceptive nerve terminals, as well as acetylcholine, norepinephrine, serotonin, and substance P.

Commonly used opioid analgesics in Oral Medicine

- Tramadol is a centrally acting analgesic whose mechanism of action is predominantly based on blockade of serotonin reuptake.
- Tramadol has been found to inhibit norepinephrine transporter function.
- Because it is only partially antagonized by naloxone, it is believed to be only a weak u-receptor agonist.
- The recommended dosage is 50- 100 mg i.m. morphine.
- Plasma half–life 4 to 6 hrs.
- Tramadol causes less respiratory depression, sedation, constipation, urinary retention, than morphine.
- Toxicity includes association with seizures, the drug is relatively contraindicated in patients with a history of epilepsy and for use with other drugs that lower the seizures threshold

- Other side effects include nausea, dizziness, but these symptoms typically abate after several days of therapy
- It surprising that no clinically significant effects on respiration or the cardiovascular system have thus far been reported
- Given the fact that the analgesic action of tramadol is largely independent of u receptor action tramadol mar serve as an adjunct with pure opioid agonist in the treatment of chronic neuropathic pain
- Tramadol (ultram) is a synthetic codeine analog that is a weak m-opioid receptor agonist
- Part of its analgesic effect is produced by inhibition of uptake of norepinephrine and serotonin
- In the treatment of mild- to – moderate pain, tramadol is as effective morphine or meperidine.
- However, for the treatment of severe or chronic, tramadol is less effective
- Tramadol is as effective as meperidine in the treatment of labour pain and may cause less neonatal respiratory depression.

Pharmacokinetics

Tramadol is 86% bio available after a single oral dose and 100% available when administered intramuscularly.

- Its affinity for the m – opioid receptor is only 1/ 6000 that of morphine.
- However, the primary O- demethylated metabolite of tramadol is two to four times as potent as the parent drug and may account for part of the analgesic effect
- Tramadol is supplied as a racemic mixture, which is more effective than either enantiomer alone. the (+) - enantiomer bind to the m-receptor and inhabits serotonin uptake
- The (+)- enantiomer inhibits norepinephrine uptake and stimulate a2 adrenergic receptors
- The compound undergoes hepatic metabolism and renal excretion, with an elimination of – life of 6 hours for tramadol and 7.5 hours for its active metabolite
- Analgesic begins within an hour of oral dosing and peaks within 2- to 3 hours
- The duration of analgesic is about 6 hrs.

- The maximum recommended daily dose is 400mg. Common side effects of tramadol include nausea, vomiting, dizziness, dry mouth, sedation, and headache.
- Respiratory depression appears to be less than with equianalgesic those of morphine. and the degree of constipation is less than that seen after equivalent dosage of codeine
- Tramadol can cause seizers and possibly exacerbate seizures in patients with predisposing factors.
- While tramadol – induced analgesia is not entirely reversible by naloxone, tramadol – induced respiratory depression can be reversed by naloxone
- However, the use of naloxone increases the risk of seizures
- Physical dependence on and abuse oof tramadol have been reported.
- Although its abuse potential is unclear, tramadol probably should be avoided in patients with history of addiction
- Because of its inhibitory effect on serotonin uptake, tramadol should not be used in patients taking monoamine oxidase inhibitors (MAO)

Use

- Tramadol is widely used for moderate to severe pain including post operative pain.
- It can be administered by mouth or by intramuscular or intravenous injection

Mechanism of action

- Tramadol works partly through an agonist effect at u receptors (Opioid action) and partly by enhancing amine (5HT and catecholamine) transmission (and hence gating mechanism) by blocking neuronal amine re-uptake.

Adverse effects

- These differ from pure opioid agonist, including less respiratory depression
- Constipation
- Abuse potential
- Diarrhea
- Abdominal pain
- Hypotension

- Psychiatric reactions
- Seizures
- Withdrawal syndromes.

Pentazocin

Exerts Many Morphene-Like Actions (analgesia, sedation, respiratory depression, nausea, decreased GI motility, it is thought to achieve its effects by stimulating receptors which are different from those that of morphine.

Dextropropoxyphene, Ethoheptazine

These two compounds are structurally related to methadone and pethidine respectively, often they are used in combination with other mild analgesics, although they have no anti pyretic, anti-tussive, or anti-inflammatory activity.

Narcotic analgesics

Codeine

Dextromoramide, dihydrocodeine

Fentanyl

Hydromorphone

Methadone

Morphine

Oxycodone

Papaveretum

Pethidine

Phenoperidine

Mode of Action

Produces analgesia and depression of associated anxiety depression of couch reflex, respiratory depression, sedation, mental clouding, euphoria, or dysphoria, miosis, CTZ stimulation, inducing vomiting or nausea, release of ADH leading to decreased urine output, release of histamine leading to flushing and constipation. Continued use produces tolerance and physical dependence –addiction TO DRUG.

Skeletal Muscle Relaxants

Introduction

- Drugs that affect skeletal muscle function include two different therapeutic groups - those used during surgical procedures and in the intensive care unit (ICU) to produce paralysis (i.e., neuromuscular blockers), and those used to reduce spasticity in a variety of painful conditions (i.e., spasmolytics).
- Neuromuscular blocking drugs interfere with transmission at the neuromuscular end plate and lack central nervous activity. These compounds are used primarily as adjuncts during general anesthesia to facilitate tracheal intubation and optimize surgical conditions while ensuring adequate ventilation.
- Drugs in the spasmolytic group have traditionally been called "centrally acting" "muscle relaxants" and are used primarily to treat chronic back pain and fibromyalgia conditions.
- Dantrolene, a spasmolytic agent that has no significant central effects and is used primarily to treat a rare anesthetic related complication, malignant hyperthermia.

Neuromuscular Blocking Drugs

History

During the 16th century, European explorers found that natives in the Amazon Basin of South America were using curare, an arrow poison that produced skeletal muscle paralysis, to kill animals. The active compound, d-tubocurarine, and its modern synthetic derivatives, have had a major influence on the practice of anesthesia and surgery and have proved useful in understanding the basic mechanisms involved in neuromuscular transmission.

Normal Neuromuscular Function

- The arrival of an action potential at the motor nerve terminal causes an influx of calcium and release of the neurotransmitter acetylcholine.
- Acetylcholine then diffuses across the synaptic cleft to activate the nicotinic receptors located on the motor end plate.
- The binding of two acetylcholine molecules to receptors causes opening of the channel. The subsequent movement of sodium and potassium is associated with a graded depolarization of the end plate membrane.

- This change in voltage is termed the motor end plate.
- The magnitude of the endplate potential is directly related to the amount of acetylcholine released. If the potential is small, the permeability and the end plate potential return to normal without an impulse being propagated from the end plate region to the rest of the muscle membrane.
- However, if the end plate potential is large, the adjacent muscle membrane is depolarized, and an action potential will be propagated along the entire muscle fiber.
- Muscle contraction is then initiated by excitation – contraction coupling.
- The released acetylcholine is quickly removed from the end plate region by both diffusion and enzymatic destruction by the local acetylcholinesterase Enzyme.

Basic Pharmacology of Neuromuscular Blocking Drugs

Chemistry

- All of the available neuromuscular blocking drugs bear a structural resemblance to acetylcholine.

- For example, succinylcholine is two acetylcholine molecules linked end to end.
- In contrast to the single linear structure of succinylcholine and other depolarizing drugs, the nondepolarizing agents (e.g., pancuronium) conceal the "double- acetylcholine" structure in one of two types of bulky, semi rigid ring systems.
- The two major families of non-depolarizing blocking drugs – the isoquinoline and steroid derivatives. Another feature common to all currently used neuromuscular blockers is the presence of one or two quaternary nitrogen's, which makes them poorly lipid – soluble and limits entry into the CNS.

Spasmolytic drugs

- Spasticity is characterized by an increase in tonic stretch reflexes and flexor muscles spasms (i.e., increased basal muscle tone) together with muscle weakness. It is often associated with spinal injury, cerebral palsy, multiple sclerosis, and stroke.
- These conditions often involve abnormal function of the bowel and bladder as well as skeletal muscle.

- The mechanisms underlying clinical Spasticity appear to involve not only the stretch reflex arc itself but also higher centers in the CNS (i.e., upper motor neuron lesion), with damage to descending pathways in the spinal cord resulting in hyper excitability of the alpha motor neurons in the cord.
- Pharmacologic therapy may ameliorate some of the symptoms of spasticity by modifying the stretch reflex arc or by interfering directly with skeletal muscle (i.e., excitation- contraction coupling).
- A variety of pharmacologic agents described as depressants of the spinal "polysynaptic" reflex arc (e.g., barbiturates [Phenobarbital] and glycerol ethers [mephensin]) have been used to treat these conditions of excess skeletal muscle tone.
- Nonspecific depression of synapses involved in the stretch reflex could reduce the desired GABAergic inhibitory activity, as well as the excitatory glutamatergic transmission.
- Currently available drugs can provide significant relief from painful muscle spasms, but they are less effective in improving meaningful function (e.g., mobility and return to work)

Diazepam

- Benzodiazepines facilitate the action of aminobutyric acid (GABA) in the central nervous system.
- Diazepam acts at GABA A synapses, and its action in reducing Spasticity is at least partly mediated in the spinal cord because it is somewhat effective in patients with cord transaction.
- Although diazepam can be used in patients with muscle spasm of almost any origin (including local muscle trauma), it also produces sedation at the doses required to reduce muscle tone
- The initial dosage is 4 mg / day, and it is gradually increased to a maximum of 60 mg /day.
- Diazepam and ketazolam (benzodiazepines) are commonly used as they have good muscle relaxant properties; they act centrally by potentiating the activity of GABA, which itself is an inhibitory neurotransmitter involved in the control of skeletal muscles.

Baclofen

- Baclofen (P-chlorphenyl –GABA) was designed to be an orally active GABA mimetic agent and is an agonist at GABAB receptors.

- Activation of these receptors by Baclofen results in hyperpolarization, probably by increased K+ conductance.
- It has been suggested that hyperpolarization causes presynaptic inhibition by reducing calcium influx and reduce the release of excitatory transmitters in both the brain and the spinal cord
- Baclofen may also reduce pain in patients with Spasticity, perhaps by inhibiting the release of substance P (neurokinin- 1) in the spinal cord.
- Baclofen is at least as effective as diazepam in reducing Spasticity and causes less sedation.
- In addition, Baclofen does not reduce overall muscle strength as much as dantrolene.
- It is rapidly and completely absorbed after oral administration and has a plasma half-life of 3-4 hrs.
- Dosage is started at 15mg twice daily, increasing as tolerated to 100mg daily.
- Adverse effects of this drug include drowsiness, however, patients become tolerant to the sedative effect with chronic administration.
- Increased seizure activity has been reported in epileptic patients therefore, withdrawal from Baclofen must be done very slowly

Other Centrally Acting Spasmolytic Drugs

Gabapentin

Is an antiepileptic that has shown considerable promise as a spasmolytic agent in several studies involving patients with multiple sclerosis.

Pregabalin

Is a newer analog of gabapentin that may also prove useful in relieving painful disorders that involve a muscle spasm component.

Progabide

Have also been found in preliminary studies to reduce Spasticity

Progabide is a GABAA and GABAB agonist and has active metabolite, including GABA itself.

Glycine

Is another inhibitory amino acid neurotransmitter that appears to possess pharmacologic activity when given orally and readily passes that blood brain barrier.

Idrocilamide and Riluzole

Are newer drugs for the treatment of amyotrophic lateral sclerosis (ALS) that appear to have spasm reducing effects possibly through inhibition of glutamatergic transmission in the central nervous system.

Botulinum Toxin

- Local facial injections of botulinum toxin are widely used for the short-term treatment (1-3 months per treatment) of wrinkles associated with aging around the eyes and mouth
- Local injection of botulinum toxin has also become a useful treatment for generalized spastic disorder (cerebral palsy)
- Most clinical studies to date have involved administration in one or two limbs, and the benefits appear to persist for weeks to several months after a single treatment.

Drugs To Treat Acute Local Muscle Spasm

A large number of less well studied, centrally acting drugs are promoted for the relief of acute muscle spasm caused by local tissue trauma or muscle strains. It has been suggested that these drugs act primarily at the level of brain stem. Carisoprodol, chlormezanone and methocarbamol are centrally acting muscle relaxants. They act predominantly within the spinal cord where they block polysynaptic reflexes. Usually, they are combined with an analgesic for use in painful conditions where muscle spasm is a factor.

Orphenadrine is a centrally acting anticholinergic drug with muscle relaxant properties.

- Carisoprodol
- Chlorophenesin
- Chlorzoxazone
- Cyclobenzaprine
- Metaxalone
- Methocarbamol, and
- Orphenadrine
- Cyclobenzaprine may be regarded as the prototype of this group

Cyclobenzaprine is structurally related to the tricyclic anti-depressant and produces anti muscarinic side effects.

- It is ineffective in treating muscle spasm due to cerebral palsy or spinal cord injury.

As a result of its strong anti-muscarinic actions, cyclobenzaprime may cause significant sedation as well as confusion and transient visual hallucinations

- The dosage of cyclobenzaprime for acute injury related muscle spasm is 20-40mg / d in divided doses orally.

Tizanidine

- Clonidine and other imidazoline compounds have a variety of effects on the CNS that are not fully understood. Among these effects is the ability to reduce muscle spasm.
- Tizanidine is a congener of clonidine that has been studied for the spasmolytic action.
- Tizanidine has significant alpha 2-adrenoceptor agonist effect, but it reduces Spasticity in experimental models at doses that cause severe cardiovascular effects than clonidine (and alpha 2- agonist-antagonist) or dexmedetomidine (a pure alpha 2 agonist).
- Neurophysiologic studies in animals and humans suggest that Tizanidine reinforces both presynaptic and post synaptic inhibition in the cord.
- It also inhibits nociceptive transmission in the spinal dorsal horn
- Clinical trials with oral Tizanidine report comparable efficacy in reliving muscle spasm to diazepam, Baclofen, and Dantrolene.

- However, Tizanidine produces a different spectrum of adverse effects, including drowsiness, hypotension, dry mouth, and asthenia.
- The dosage requirement varies markedly among patients and individual dosage titration is necessary to achieve an optimal clinical effect
- Brand names (zanaflex, sirdalud) is a drug that is used as a muscle relaxant
- It is a centrally acting (alpha) α 2 adrenergic agonist
- It is used to treat the spasm, cramping and lightness of muscles caused by medical problems such as multiple sclerosis, spastic diplegia, back pain, or certain other injuries to the spine or CNS.
- It is also prescribed off label for migraine headaches, as a sleep aid and as an anti-convulsant
- It is also prescribed for some symptoms of fibro myalgia
- Tizanidine has been found to be as effective as other anti-spasmodic drugs and had superior tolerability than Baclofen and diazepam.
- Tizanidine may cause hypotension, caution is advised when it is used in patients who had a history of orthostatic hypotension

- Use caution with this drug as it can be very strong even at the 2mg dose. Also use caution when switching from gel cap to tablet from and vice versa.

Availability

- Tizanidine is supplied as 2 and 4 mg tablets for oral administration, and in gel cap form in doses of 2mg, 4mg and 6mg.
- The tablets are composed of the active ingredient, Tizanidine hydrochloride (2.288 mg equivalent to 2mg Tizanidine base and 4.576 mg equivalent to 4 mg Tizanidine base.
- Inactive ingredients silicon dioxide colloidal and anhydrous lactose.

Side effects

- Feeling light headed, fainting, slow heart rate.
- Hallucinations, confusion, unusual thoughts or behavior.
- Nausea, stomach pain, low fever, loss of appetite, dark urine, clay-colored stools, Jaundice (yellowing of the skin or eyes)
- Burning / painful micturition.

Less Serious Tizanidine Side Effects

- Drowsiness or dizziness
- Feeling nervous or anxious
- Numbness or tingling
- Stomach pain, diarrhea, constipation
- Vomiting
- Fever
- Dry mouth
- Muscle weakness, back pain
- Increased muscle tone or spasms
- Sweating or skin rashes

Tizanidine dosing Information

Usual Adult Dose for Muscle Spasm-

- The initial dose of Tizanidine recommended for this patient with increase muscle tone associated with Spasticity related to multiple sclerosis of spinal cord injury is 4mg orally, once a day. The dose of Tizanidine may be repeated as needed at 6-8 hourly intervals to a maximum dose of three doses / 24 hrs.

- The dose may be gradually increased (every 4-7 days) in increments of 1-2 mg until desired response is attained.
- The manufacturer recommends that total daily dose should not exceed 36 mg. additionally, the use of single doses greater than 12 mg is not recommended starting at a lower dose and titrating upwards minimizes the risk for adverse effects.
- Experience with single dose greater than 8 mg and total daily dose greater than 24 mg is limited. Effects appear to be dose related gradually diminish within 3-6 hrs. after a dose. Use must be individualized and directed at times and activities where benefit is most important.

Usual Geriatric Dose for Muscle Spasm-

- In geriatric patients, a starting dose of 2mg orally once a day may be appropriate

Interactions

- Concomitant use of Tizanidine and moderate or potent CYP1A2 Inhibitors is contraindicated.
- Concomitant use of Tizanidine with fluvoxamine, a potent CYP1A2 inhibitor in man, resulted in a 33-fold increases in the

Tizanidine AUC (plasma drug concentration –time curve) by fluvoxamine.

What Other Drugs Will Affect Tizanidine?

- Acyclovir (Zovirax)
- Cimitidine (Tagamet)
- Famotidine (Pepcid)
- Ticlopidine (Ticlid)
- Zileuton (zyflo)
- Birth control pills
- **Antibiotics** such as enoxacin (penetrex), gatifloxacin (Tequin), levofloxacin, (Levaquin), lomefloxacin (maxaquin), moxifloxacin (Avelox), ofloxacin (Floxin), sparfloxacin (Zagam), trovafloxacin (Trovan), or Norfloxacin (noroxin)
- **Blood pressure medications** such as clonidine (Catapres), guanabenz (Wytensin), guanfacine (Tenex) or methyldopa (Aldomet).
- **Heart rhythm medications** such as amiodarone (cordarone, Peecerone), mexiletine (Mexitil), propafenone (Rhythmol), and verapamil (Calan, Covera, Isoptin).

References

6. Goodman and Gilmans, The pharmacological basis of therapeutic - 11th Ed (2006) by Kaball.
7. Basic and clinical pharmacology 11th Ed Bertram G. Katzung, Susan B Masters, Anthony J Trevor
8. Essential of medical pharmacology K D Tripathi 6th edition
9. The Dental clinics of North America Drugs Prescribed to Dental patients, Vol 38, no 4, Oct 1994.
10. A textbook of clinical pharmacology and therapeutics, 5th ed, james M ritter
11. Oral medicine diagnosis and treatment Burkets 10th Ed
12. www.scielo.isciii.es - use of nonsteroidal ant inflammatory drugs in dental practice
13. www.ada.org - oral analgesics for acute dental pain
14. www.nps.org.au-medical management of dental and oral pain
15. www.webmd.com - drugs used in dentistry's
16. www.clevelandclinic.org - dentistry medication – Cleveland Clinic.

Index